Keeping My Faith While Saving My Mind

Memoirs of Overcoming Traumas

SHULANDA J. HASTINGS

Copyright © 2017 Shulanda J. Hastings/SJHastings

All rights reserved.

ISBN-13: 978-1534697003
ISBN-10: 1534697004

DEDICATION

I dedicate this book to my beloved brother, Marchello L. Johnson, whose life and legacy has contributed so greatly to mine.   As long as I breathe, I shall never forget you and will always be your voice.

CONTENTS

	Acknowledgments	i
1	Chastity Defiled	1
2	Path to Restoration	11
3	Closer than a Brother	21
4	Barriers to Acceptance	29
5	The Master's Touch	41
6	Walking in Faith	52
7	Leading While Bleeding	61
8	The Silent Killer	74
9	Keeping My Faith	84
10	Saving My Mind	94

ACKNOWLEDGEMENTS

I must first give honor to Jesus Christ, my Lord and personal Savior who has been a constant anchor in my life.

To every intercessor who has prayed for me during this journey of my life and throughout the process of birthing this book of memoirs.

To every person who continues to fight the battle to live life to its fullest, rather than just exist, there is hope.

INTRODUCTION

"For I know the plans I have for you," declares the LORD, "plans to prosper you and not to harm you, plans to give you hope and a future." – Jeremiah 29:11

Life is indeed a journey. The destination only completely known to the Designer, the God of all creation. But if we the creation accept the invitation to His intimacy, we are privileged to gain direction and insight of our purpose in life. This allows the heart of hope to continue beating forward so that we do not become stagnate in our present or held captive by our past. Because on this journey of life there will be challenging days, tragic events and internal conflicts that will cause us to reach out to the One who can make sense out of chaos; every traumatizing occurrence.

Trauma: "would be considered a situation beyond control, one that shakes a person to the core. A trauma can lead to mental disorders or to suicide. Recovery is often slow; flashbacks are common…Traumatic events overwhelm the person's ordinary adapting or coping mechanisms to life".[i]

This book of memoirs is about real events that have

occurred in my life during childhood, adolescent and single adult years. Some events I have shared with confidants and others have been shared openly through my advocacy or ministry platforms. However, these memoirs also include intimate details of my life that are revealed publicly for the very first time. I must forewarn that although I have intentionally written this book to be an easy read, depending on your personal experiences you might find some passages to be difficult to digest. There are sensitive topics, yet relevant and transparent issues that are discussed not only because they have happened to me, but to so many others who have silenced them out of fear. And my ultimate goal is to eradicate the fear and by being a voice.

Keeping My Faith While Saving My Mind; Memoirs of Overcoming Traumas is presented in a coupled format. The first chapter of each section includes the narrative version of my memoir and it is directly followed by a post-reflective chapter that is comprised of educational, encouraging and insightful readings. Because life has positioned me as an expert and I have served in leading advocacy positions, a particular tone and terminology is used throughout this book. However, I do not write this from any particular professional's perspective, but rather from a personal one.

Penning these memoirs was indeed challenging for me to write. I experienced major hurdles and setbacks while writing and publishing this book. In fact, I know that out of all of my previous and post writings, it will be the work that I consider the most significant and necessary. In my heart, it feels long overdue. But because I know that God's timing is perfect it is being released at the appointed time. Even so, because of the enemy's skewed peak view of my destiny I know he has been strategically fighting to abort this project from being birthed. Nevertheless, I trust the entire process was worth the anticipated outcome.

It is my hope that this book will ultimately contribute to breaking the barrier of silence that hinders the process of overcoming traumatic events specifically among believers. It is my prayer that this book will help heal many of you on an individual level, enhance your ministries to help those hurting who are in need of healing and deliverance, causing all to live a victorious life rooted in faith.

Keeping My Faith

1 CHASTITY DEFILED

"For I will restore health to you, and your wounds I will heal, declares the LORD." - Jeremiah 30:17, ESV

Children have to deal with different forms of trauma causing innocence to be a rare commodity. Yet, I believe all good parents want to preserve this virtue for their children. As adults, we seem to be losing this battle in protecting our children, this generation from being robbed of their innocent childhood experiences. As Christians, we can do a better job in standing our ground for what we value and be a voice for the small voices depending on us.

Do you know how many broken families are in your congregation right now? Do you know how many shameful family secrets are being kept every Sunday as you minister through music in your choir? Do you know how many girls are hurting inside every time you try to convince them to be a part of your youth ministry only led by male leaders? Unfortunately, there are too many youth within your church who are currently dealing with a traumatizing crisis situation.

Crisis situations occur every day, every hour, every minute. Although we hear of traumatic experiences occurring among children, it is often when these children have grown to adults that we hear their stories. As a Christian counselor, I have worked with many people who suffer from the painful traumas that occurred in their childhood. For most of them, I was the first to hear their stories. Allow me to share unpleasant experiences of mine that are considered a norm in many families.

As a little girl growing up in the rural of Clarksdale, Mississippi, my Grandmother did her best to raise me in the church and teach me about God. She was in charge of opening and closing the physical doors of our church, and every time she did, her entire household accompanied her. She worked hard to send all of us to a private school where I attended until a lack of funding resulted in the doors to be permanently closed.

Craving a change from Southern life, all of my Grandmother's children decided to move to California for a fresh start. Her first born and oldest daughter, my mother, was the first to relocate. Initially left behind, I was eager to make the transition with my aunts and uncles. It had been quite some time since I had seen my brothers and I looked forward to the opportunity to see them everyday and make great long lasting memories. But it didn't quite work out that way.

The first day we arrived in California, we went by my mother's home. I recall it like it was yesterday. Already star struck by all the glamour we passed to get to Long Beach, I nearly jumped out of a moving car to hurry inside my mother's one bedroom apartment. I vastly anticipated seeing my younger brother Marchello who was seven at the time. Being the oldest, we were the closest out of our four siblings. After we all had mingled for a couple of hours, my uncles and aunts were preparing to leave to check on their newly rented house. Under the impression I would be living with my mother, I rushed to the car to get my things. I was sadly mistaken. My mother wasn't as elated to see me as I was to see them. Therefore, I lived with my uncle, my mother's brother.

About a year later, my uncle had to relocate his family to the Oakland area due to his job. Since I was still in school, he and my mother made an arrangement for me to live with her. Again excited about the chance to live with my brothers, I had no complaints. I just didn't know how the new living arrangement would forever change my life.

By this time, my mother had upgraded to a two bedroom apartment and had a new live in boyfriend. I was 11-years-old when I moved in with them and was still sheltered and protected by the innocence in which my Grandmother had raised me. I had never witnessed unmarried people living together. I had never been around a man in a household setting who wasn't any kin to me. But I was taught to respect all adults and I did.

In the beginning, my mother's boyfriend appeared to be nice. And that was just it. He was nice to me. He made my brothers practically slave around our apartment doing chores. When I would attempt to help them, he forbade it. During our grocery store visits, he would always buy me candy, never permitting them to select any treats. My mother yielded to his actions. Whether out of fear or submission, I don't know. He would also humiliate her, but would try to do it in a joking way. Pretty soon, things turned into no joking matter.

On a particular night after we all had finished watching a sequence of television shows, everyone departed for bed. I was the last one in the bathroom and after I came out, my mother's boyfriend was still up in the living room. He called for me to join him on the sofa and watch television with him. Uncomfortable, I told him I was sleepy and wanted to go to bed. He insisted that I stay up for a little while longer.

These particular nights started with small talk. He pretended to be interested in my school and social life. He kept the living room completely dark. The only light came from the television. The nights would end with him making me give him a massage that would lead to him guiding my hand to his private parts. I didn't understand why he was doing that to me. He made it seem as though it was naturally expected of me. I wanted to protect my brothers. As long as I kept quiet, he seemed to treat them better. Because my mother and I never connected and she always made me feel as though I was an inconvenience, I never disclosed any of this to her. So this continued up until one night.

One night, my brother Marchello got up to use the bathroom and he heard the television still on in the living room. Upon his entrance, he walked in on my mother's boyfriend molesting me. Since it was still dark in the room, I didn't know what he had seen. But my mother's boyfriend quickly told him to go back to bed. Reluctantly, he did. I used the momentary interruption as a way of escape. Hastily, I got up from the sofa and followed my brother into the bedroom that all of my siblings and I shared.

Our room was quiet. As I laid alone in my bed, all I could hear was the sound of my sniffles. No matter how much I tried to silence them, it didn't hide the fact that I was uncontrollably crying. I thought I was the only one up in the room. I wondered if my brother had seen anything. It was only until he spoke that it was confirmed that he had.

"How long has he been doing that?" he asked.

My heart had to have skipped a beat. In one way, I was relieved that someone knew. But at the same time, I knew the consequences of my brother knowing. Although three years younger than I, Marchello considered himself my big brother. We stayed up mostly all that night. After I explained all that had been going on to him, I had to spend time convincing him not to confront our mother's boyfriend. But he only agreed on one condition: that we tell our aunt. He too knew that telling our mother wouldn't make a big difference. So the next day, we devised a plan to get on the bus in north Long Beach, where we lived, and rode it back to the eastside where my aunt resided.

My brother supported me throughout the entire process of telling our aunt, talking to the police and even testifying on my behalf. My mother's boyfriend who was convicted, had surprisingly been wanted in another state for doing the same thing. Despite the justice the law gave me, I was still scarred. I had been violated. And perhaps I could have dealt with it better had my mother showed some support. Even after her boyfriend was sentenced to jail, she visited him. My uncle had to confront her about doing so and even taking down the pictures that she still had in our apartment of him. Things were never again the same. I longed for my Grandmother. I missed my life in Mississippi. Once summer arrived, I went back to the

South.

I thought I was returning to a safe place. And as always at my Grandmother's house, it was. But that summer she allowed me to do something that she never would have agreed to: spend a week at another one of my aunts house in Itta Bena, Mississippi, outside of Greenwood. My Grandmother was very particular about me staying with others on her watch. It was because of a potential incident like the one in California that she wanted to prevent. But I wanted to spend time with my male cousin, who was as close to me as my brother. He was attending a youth camp for all ages and I wanted to attend too. I craved to feel like a child again. Grandmother must have felt sympathetic to what I had just experienced, so she hesitantly agreed. How I wish she would have stood her ground.

The environment in Itta Bena was not one that I needed to be exposed to. As my mother, my aunt kept an open house. Any and everyone could walk in and out and they pretty much did. The normal traffic consisted of adults; married couples coming over for a game of spades, married couples coming over without their spouses to meet with their nighttime lovers, the community alcoholics, the ladies of the evenings. It was pretty much a hotel and night club combined into one. But this was mostly the norm for every household in the small town during that time. I thought I had seen a lot in California, but had no idea this type of lifestyle existed in my own backyard in Mississippi!

One day during a typical house gathering, a 29-year-old family friend asked me, a then 12-year-old to do something totally out of the ordinary, especially for me.

"Pretty girl," he said sitting at the round table where a card game and drinking was going on. "Will you call my wife and tell her I am going to be late coming home?"

At first, I didn't think he was serious. But he was. After giving a confused look to my aunt, she instructed me to do so. Needless to say, that was the most awkward conversation I ever had to have. But before the end of my stay, my childhood innocence would be further tainted.

The following afternoon, this same man stopped by my aunt's house. My cousins and I were there alone. After he generously sent them walking to the store, he then had me at the house by myself. I went in my aunt's room to watch television to leave him in the living room by himself. I prayed that my cousins would hurry back, but they were little boys. They were bound to make stops along the way. So I prayed that someone would come by and give a surprise visit; preferably, a woman. Neither hopeful wish happened. And soon, the 29-year-old married man, came into my aunt's room.

Everything happened so fast. Unfortunately, it was unlike the incident I had experienced with my mother's boyfriend who had limited his violation to molestation. This time I had been sexually assaulted and had blood stained evidence left behind. I was in shock. I couldn't move mentally or physically. After he finished, he simply got up, went back in the living room and started watching television. After my aunt's cruel response that insinuated that I was now considered a woman after my California incident and this is what's expected of women, I never told any one about the incident until I was an adult.

2 PATH TO RESTORATION

Sexual abuse: Sexual abuse occurs whenever a child is exploited by an older person for the satisfaction of the abuser's needs; it consists of any sexual activity (visual, verbal, or physical) engaged in without consent. The child is considered unable to consent because of developmental immaturity.[ii]

Millions of children have been abused either verbally, physically or sexually. Some of these cases have been reported and others have not. Christian families are not exempt from these statistics. In some cases, many abusers are in the homes of Christian families; therefore, embedded within our local churches. Does this mean that God is not present in these families? No, it does not. The enemy's intent is to kill, steal and destroy families (ref. John 10:10). When families are broken and divided, they are easily cursed. But curses can be reversed. And blessings can be restored. Whether you are a woman in need of restoring from a childhood abuse, currently mentoring a child or ministering to a young lady who has been abused, let's journey the Path to Restoration.

Intervention

There is an unspoken code of protection in many families; silence. I have learned that the logic behind it is protection; protection from ridicule, protection from a scandal. This code is in place to protect the family, but does not help the victims; those that continue to suffer due to the sacrifice they make on behalf of their loved ones. Because children are easily influenced by adults, they too quickly learn this unspoken code. As a result, child abuse situations continue and children never receive the help and healing that is required.

<u>Breaking the Silence</u>

Let's revisit my child abuse experiences. In a way, silence was used as an enabling tool. That does not suggest it was my fault or any child that has been on the receiving end of such violation. But silence is a tool that perpetrators use in order to continue their violent acts. In the first abusive incident that involved my mother's boyfriend, he depended on me not saying anything. He knew there was a disconnect in the relationship with my mother and used it to manipulate his plan. It was only until silence was broken that his abuse towards me stopped.

Luke 8:17 informs us that, "For all that is secret will eventually be brought into the open, and everything that is concealed will be brought to light and made known to all" (NLT). God does not want acts of abuse or any act that hurts His creation, His children to be kept hidden. God does not expect us to be a sacrifice for darkness. Our Father does not want us to keep our pains a secret, even if they are going to expose or bring shame to those we love. He wants us to break the silence so that we can get help.

Getting Help

Children are often abused by those they know and that have easy access to them. Therefore, these abusers are also close acquaintances to the family or even relatives themselves. This makes it difficult to reach out to a trusted family member when such trust has already been broken. My brother was my confidant. He did not even consider keeping my molestation a secret. In fact, he quickly orchestrated a plan for me to get help so that our mother's boyfriend could be exposed. What bravery and boldness from a then eight-year-old.

Unfortunately, most children do not feel as though they have a special person to confide in within their families. If the abuser is mom's significant other, as in my case, they struggle with the fear of their mother not believing them. If it is a close friend or distant relative in the family, as in my second story, the environment created by the adults does not make the child feel secure in opening up. This is where other outlets have to serve as safe places for children to break their silence and get help.

As I will share later in chapter eight, youth sometimes find it easier to open up to strangers or outsiders about such private incidents. They might find it more comfortable talking to a teacher, school counselor, mentor or minister. School educators and administrators are trained to identify types of abuse and understand their duty to report. The church was designed to be a more prominent safe haven than school. However, it is the church that is more relaxed in its approach to handling abuse in families. Why do you think this is?

You have probably guessed it. The same code of protection in families is embedded in church families. Certainly the church does not want to protect abusers; we already know that is not God's will. But how this code is at work in our local congregations is that there is: (1) Lack of Responsibility, (2) Lack of Understanding, and (3) Lack of Training.

1. Lack of Responsibility. While ministering at various churches either through evangelistic outreach or mental health advocacy, common responses that I hear that are barriers for children and even adults that are in abusive situations not receiving help boils down to a lack of responsibility. *That's not my place to get involved in their business. All I can do is pray for them. That is for the leaders or authorities to handle.*

There is a passive approach taken in our churches in regards to people with issues. Yes, the church. The very place that is meant to be the connecting point to the Great Burden Bearer. Millions of people bring their issues every week to a place for help and the members are confused about their authority and responsibility to help them. So either out of tradition or ignorance or both, they simply choose to pacify the problem.

2. Lack of Understanding. "..therefore get wisdom: and with all thy getting get understanding" (Proverbs 4:7, KJV). This is a prominent barrier to intervention and will be discussed throughout this book. Now of course those being abused wonder why they are being abused. As a child, I wondered why my mother's boyfriend and my aunt's friend of the family did what they did to me. I pondered on this question during their acts of sexual abuse, immediately afterwards and throughout my life. As relevant as this question is for closure, it is not the lack of understanding that I'm referring to.

As believers, naturally we are taught the importance of prayer. And without a doubt, prayer is one of our most powerful weapons. Pardon my tone, but the church has confused using prayer as a weapon against the enemy with prayer as an excuse not to do any work. For example, a woman who goes to a church for help after being sexually abused needs to be comforted through prayer and reminded that God still loves her. That God wants to restore her. But that is not where ministry ends.

Allow me to share a true story with you. I once visited a church for their mid-week service. It was your typical Bible study and in this case allowed for an intimate fellowship among attendees. It had been a great teaching message and as the pastor was about to give the benediction, he asked for any prayer requests. Surprisingly, among those with a request was a young adult woman. She could barely articulate her prayer request. It was very evident that she was in emotional distress. She was uncontrollably crying and shaking as she told those in attendance a story that was unexpected at that moment.

The very day before this young lady had been violated by a man who forced his way into her apartment. Those in attendance at the Bible study were the first she told her story to. This particular church was the only local support system that she had because all of her family lived in other states. She had not notified her family about the incident or the authorities. Prior to coming to the church, she had been driving around because she was fearful to return to her apartment, thinking her sexual abuser would come back to her home. The place she felt comfortable to come to for help, more comfortable than picking up the phone to call her family was her church. What was the church's response?

The pastor added her request to the collective prayer,

assigned an intercessor to pray with her immediately after service and walked back to his office. As a crisis counselor who has handled calls for sexual assault centers, all kind of thoughts were streaming through my mind. I wondered about her safety and emotional state. I thought about the 48-72 hour window to examine victims to capture any remaining evidence in the event she chooses to file charges.

Although reluctant to approach her because I was a visiting minister and the pastor had already set the order, I did so anyway. She was surrounded by ladies; some praying and others preying. By the time I had an opportunity to speak with her, she was still sobbing. I briefly spoke words of encouragement in her ear as I gave her an extended hug and left my card with her, hoping she would reach out. But relating to her situation, I knew the odds of her contacting me were slim to none. Therefore, I followed up with the pastor the next day. He returned my call days after and unsurprisingly, had not made any contact with his member and appeared nonchalant about doing so.

You might be having unpleasant thoughts towards the pastor as I initially did, but I had to discern some hard truths. First, I don't think that the pastor was as unconcerned about what to do as it appeared he was. Like many other pastors, I believe it was his lack of understanding or knowledge about what to do and his obligation to do it. This brings me to my next point.

3. Lack of Training. Most ministers and spiritual leaders receive some formal training either through seminary or their church's affiliated denomination. However, there aren't many clergy who have a background or any formal training in counseling. Which is very unfortunate when you consider the platform they have and the role they play in their communities. Even so, many churches are fortunate enough to have professionals in the field of mental health, social work and counseling. The misfortune is that they are not utilized. I often hear the complaints from both faith-based and secular counselors how they have a difficult time working with churches and pastors. I, myself, can attest to this.

A trained minister would know that whether or not he or she does not have the expertise in helping someone does not mean they are not obligated to help connect the person to resources. A school teacher may or may not be trained in social work or criminal justice, but he or she understands the obligation of their duty to report abuse. This is the step in intervention that we want to reach.

<u>Stopping the Violation</u>

A person being abused can not start the process to healing until they are no longer being abused. A firefighter can not stop a person from burning inside a house by simply taking them to a different room. They need to be rescued from the burning building. Thankfully, the ongoing molestation that I was in stopped when my silence was broken and I got help to remove my mother's boyfriend from my environment. But my one time childhood rape incident was kept silent until my adulthood. And this caused damage to my trust in men and women. Men for the obvious reason and with women because women who were suppose to be close to me allowed me to be violated. I went through different prolonged stages of pain and suffering, as victims do. As this journey continues, you will gain a glimpse of the physical, emotional, cognitive, relational and spiritual effects of not just my abuse, but that of the so many others in your churches.

3 CLOSER THAN A BROTHER

"The LORD is close to the brokenhearted and saves those who are crushed in spirit." - Psalms 34: 18, NIV.

Every person will experience grief at some point in life. Some more often than others. Regardless of the number of times we deal with the death of a loved one, each experience nearly feels like the first time. It is also the manner and method by which one dies that effects how we grieve. If someone has been diagnosed with a terminal illness, seldom are we caught off guard by their death. But when someone has been in an accident or death occurred in a tragic way, it can be a very difficult pill to swallow. I will share by far the most painful grievance that I have ever experienced.

It is frequently quoted, that "a picture is worth a thousand words." As I stare at the last picture taken with my brother, this declaration holds truth. Eyes can easily rest on the background of flowers clothed by thorns and vines in the country, but my mind simmers on the compelling story being told by the invisible thorns; the unspoken words. Twenty years have passed since this photograph was captured. As the first time I saw it; instantly, I recapitulate the day that would forever change my life. I have played out hundreds of scenarios. I have probed a million questions. The outcome relentlessly remains the same: My brother, dead from suicide, at age 15.

He was the cheerful one, always full of laughter and enjoying life with his carefree spirit. He was my diary. I confided in him about everything; my dreams and my fears. I reciprocated the same trust to him. Our Grandmother raised me; therefore, we resided in different states. I cherished the rare weekends and random summers we spent together. The distance that divided us was no challenge to the bond we shared.

Recalling the scarred memory that day started with so much excitement. It was the day that every high school student anticipates; graduation! Most of my relatives had to travel from out of town, including my mother and siblings.

"Can we take a ride in your car?" My brother asked ten minutes after they drove up. They arrived at Grandmother's house hours late and I was due at commencement in 45 minutes.

"I really want to, but I have to be on time for lineup. We can take a ride before you all leave tomorrow." I assured him. My plan was to celebrate with him and my cousins over the weekend and my classmates over the summer, before leaving for college. Unfortunately, things didn't go as expected.

My mother left before my brother and I could take the promised joy ride. Although disappointed, I counted on having the entire summer for an opportunity to spend with him. Two weeks after graduation, my aunt came to my job 30 minutes prior to the end of my shift.

"I have something to tell you" she barely got out. Seconds later, the tears flowed down. "Mar, Marchello is dead. He hurt himself." I heard her words, but refused to comprehend them so I continued working.

It took me weeks to *accept* what had happened and

years before I could continue through the grieving process. Only until I had taken a psychology course did I realize my reactions, thoughts and feelings were actually considered normal. However, no college professor, psychologist or pastor could adequately explain the pain that I experienced after that day. Losing my brother was shattering enough, but to lose him to suicide was an even greater blow, especially for me. I was the one that had battled with depression. My brother was my protector and the one that helped me through what appeared to be the darkest times in my life. He was my voice when I couldn't verbalize my pain. The one time he needed me I couldn't be there for him. Why had God given me such a thorn to bear?

Living Inside a Box

For seven years, I struggled with depression. My family didn't understand my grief. I was often told to *just let it go* and *just move on*. But I couldn't. My church family told me that I wasn't praying enough to God or activating my faith. But I was. They didn't see me crying out to God every night, throughout the night. They didn't understand my pain. They didn't know how it felt to struggle to go to sleep at night and wake up every morning dreading that I lived to see another day. A new day wasn't a blessing for me. It was the reality of having to repeat the same cycle over again. I often described it as the *cardboard box analogy*.

Imagine that you are placed inside a cardboard box only big enough to fit your body measurements while in a sitting position. No extra space. Only a hole in one corner about the size of a quarter, allowing you just enough oxygen to survive. In order to keep breathing, you have to keep your nose close to the hole that also serves as a peephole. This hole is your sole connection to the world. You are able to gain a glimpse of people walking pass your box; talking, laughing and enjoying their lives. They aren't aware that you are inside. They don't know that you are trapped inside of your box. The reality is you are not physically bound. It is a cardboard box that only requires you to push your way out. But because you are mentally confined, you are content with merely existing inside of your box than to take a risk and live on the outside with the rest of the world.

I lived inside of my own mental cardboard box for seven consecutive years. For 84 months I merely existed and struggled with the decision to barely keep breathing or to break free. Right after learning that my 15-year-old brother had died by suicide two weeks after my high school graduation, I started the darkest cycle of my life. A cycle that would seasonally repeat itself.

I was scheduled to start college that fall. But it was the day that my brother's body arrived in Mississippi to be buried that I left to attend my college orientation that summer. To this day, I wonder if attending his burial service would have given me better closure. My family's reasoning for my absence was that Marchello would not have wanted me to stop living my life. And since attending college was a part of that plan, he would have wanted me to be present for my orientation. My body was in Oxford that week and the years to follow, but my heart and mind remained in Clarksdale, which was the last place I saw my brother alive and his final resting place.

Before allowing me to be away from home on my own for the first time, there should have been a preventative plan established. I didn't receive any grief counseling. Really, there was no support system in place. I wasn't allowed to talk about what had happened. And when I tried to do so, I was quickly silenced and the conversation was changed. My Grandmother even took down all of my brother's pictures and boxed them up. It was as if his life had never existed. There was no outlet to express what I was feeling and trying to process. I didn't personally know of anyone ever successfully completing a suicide attempt. Honestly, up until that point my culture taught me that two classes of people did not even think about taking their lives: black people and church folks.

That week of orientation was so challenging for me. And to add to my stress, I had to deal with my grief among complete strangers who had no clue what had happened to me. I literally went through the motions. If it wasn't for an assigned roommate who became a friend, I wouldn't have had any classes for the fall. Even so, it was just as if I did not. Before the completion of my Freshman year, I was in a severe suicidal state.

By this time, my family was forced to intervene. The college counseling center tried to explain to them how serious my condition had progressed. They were advised to get me professional help. This time they did reluctantly pursue treatment. But I didn't understand what was going on with me either. I was petrified. The one person I would confide in was now gone. All kind of thoughts were constantly clouding my mind. No counseling or therapy session during that time would work for me. I wasn't free to describe the issues I was dealing with. I felt like everyone thought I was now some kind of disease. To me, I was now treated like an alien. My college classmates soon branded me as the "crazy" girl and my family wasn't interested in me going to counseling to get real help; rather, to hurry up and 'fix' the problem that was causing them ridicule. This environment became my norm for the next couple of years.

4 BARRIERS TO ACCEPTANCE

Grief: "Intense emotional suffering caused by a loss".[iii]

Every time it seemed that I was making progress and moving forward, the enemy would attack my mind. He would constantly remind me how I had lost the closest person to me on earth. And when the one closest to you is physically gone, it is quite difficult to connect with those who remain or even the One who is omnipresent.

I had to learn through a period of long-suffering that there really is someone closer than a brother. And in order to get through those dark nights and days, I had to call Him many things. I had to believe and trust God to be my Comforter when no one else could comfort me. I had to depend on Jesus to be my Healer when no one understood my heart was broken. I truly learned that He "…saves those who are crushed in spirit" (Psalms 34: 18, NIV). In Hebrew, the word saves means to rescue, deliver and save from guilt. And this is what God did for me. He saved, delivered and rescued me from myself. But it was a process.

Unhealthy Grieving

Some of you are being processed right now. Many of you are helping others or trying to research ways to help others go through a process. We all have experienced losing something or someone that we love or treasure. When that person is lost in a tragic way, it can be more difficult to comprehend. As difficult as grief is, it is necessary and healthy. Unfortunately, as reflected in my situation, there are barriers that can cause it to be an unhealthy process.

When you lose a parent, sibling or child there is a void that lingers like a prolonged throbbing pain from a needle insertion. The pain is suppose to numb itself, but for some reason it won't. Those who experience bereavement of a loved one are always reminded of God, the Holy Spirit, who comforts. He comforts us in troubling times (2 Corinthians 1:4) and when we are grieving (John

16:20). And to know that God has promised to "never leave you nor forsake you" (Deuteronomy 31:6) is reassuring when there is a void that seems impossible to be filled.

Stages of Grief

Outlined below are the five basic stages of grief that was first introduced by renowned psychiatrist Elisabeth Kubler-Ross:[iv] My summarized definition has been added:

1. **Denial.** The first reaction to learning of terminal illness or death of a cherished loved is to deny the reality of the situation.
2. **Anger.** Bereaved individuals find themselves being angry with others.
3. **Bargaining.** In this stage, those grieving try to negotiate the death or bargain with God for more time or to change the outcome.
4. **Depression.** Those grieving go through a period of sadness that causes depression. They want to blame themselves for not being able to keep their loved ones alive.
5. **Acceptance.** This important stage, the bereaved accepts the death of their loved one. They reconnect with reality and work towards moving

forward, living their lives.

Remember that grief is a healthy emotion. It becomes unhealthy when the stages of grief have become stagnate for the bereaved. This causes a barrier to acceptance. This then requires an intervention to take place so that the person can receive help in taking the steps through the grieving process. In my case, I needed help maneuvering through the general stages.

Denial and Isolation. From the moment I heard my aunt tell me of my brother's death, I used denial as a defense mechanism. I certainly did not process the fact that she told me he had committed suicide. Instead of showing the emotion that my family expected, I continued the activity I was involved in. Afterwards, I went through the motions of gathering with family and attending the memorial service. My denial continued and I isolated myself from my family and eventually friends. My college dorm and later apartment became my place of refuge. Everywhere I lived I made sure that all of my windows were covered and curtains did not suffice. There had to be black poster boards covering the windows that had dark colored curtains draped over them restricting any light to shine in and restraining me from connecting with the outside world. Isolation was one of my most difficult barriers.

Anger. In a *normal* death situation the bereaved usually find themselves being angry at the loved one that has left them. I felt this towards my brother for a brief moment. But my anger was mostly directed towards myself. I was angry that I did not see that my brother needed help. I was angry that I was unable to recognize that he was feeling depressed. I was angry that I was not able to save him from such a familiar pain. I was his big sister and I had failed him. My anger soon shifted to family members. It was easy to be angry with my mother because of our disconnected relationship. But I blamed her for allowing my brother to die on her watch. I blamed her for aborting my future memories with my brother. Eventually, I grew angry with God. I couldn't understand why He allowed it to happen. Anger leads to bitterness. God tells us in Ephesians 4:31, "Let all bitterness and wrath and anger and clamor and slander be put away from you along with all malice."

Bargaining. When we feel helpless, we feel a need to want to be in control. This overlapped during my stage of anger. I had many, "If only…" moments with myself and

God. This was a challenging stage for me because my last conversation with my brother consisted of bargaining that was accompanied by a promise. My brother wanted to go joy riding and since time was conflicting, I told him that we could go later. I had planned to take him riding in my car, but they left before I had the chance. This made me repeat my stage of anger because I was angry that I did not deliver on my promise and again, I blamed my mother for not allowing me to keep that promise by deciding to leave early. I needed someone to blame. If a person is killed by someone else, whether in a car accident or crime, at least there is someone to blame. My brother's life was lost to suicide. I couldn't blame him for his pain or mental condition that he found himself in. There was no one else to blame for his death and this reality did not give me the closure that I desperately desired and needed.

Depression. Without a doubt, this was my longest and most challenging stage in the grieving process. Depression is a normal response to grief, but it is abnormal for it to last seven years. In fact, when depression lasts more than a few days, especially a couple of weeks, it has transitioned to a clinical stage of depression.[v] This means that even though this area of darkness is one that the enemy uses against even God's people, psychological intervention has to occur. A treatment plan has to be implemented. Did this happen imminently in my situation? No. It was a long process. And as piercing as the following statement is going to sting, faith and family were heavy barriers to my getting help. If you are among my targeted Christian audience, or a family-oriented person reading this, you are probably criticizing that statement. Being a Christian believer myself, I understand. But the truth is this was my truth during that difficult time. The truth is this is the reality for many others that have experienced and are struggling with the similar depression that I did: keeping their faith, while *losing their minds*. Allow me to elaborate on this a little further before going to the final grief stage.

As an adolescent, I did not have much experience with grief. As a matter of fact, prior to my brother, the only other close relative's death that I had mourned was my great grandmother, my maternal grandmother's mother. My brother was the first person I knew to lose his life to suicide. Add this crisis to the normal stressors I was expected to experience as an adolescent and college student. My family could not help me in the way I needed. It is not that they did not want to, but do you remember the unspoken code I mentioned in the previous chapter? This code of silence existed in my family. I was taught not to tell outsiders family business, which is a basic universal ground rule for families. And I believe this is okay when you view it from the perspective of family loyalty that coincides with trust. But when it crosses the boundaries of assisting family members to get help, this is when it should be unambiguously clear there is an exception to the rule.

My connection to my brother was through my family. Since we lived in different states, I didn't know his friends. Therefore, I had no one to discuss him with. No one to share memories of him with. There was another code in my family that is also in the majority of African-American families; *black people don't go to therapy and nor do we kill ourselves.* So where did this leave me to go for help? The church.

Having been reared in the church, confessed Christ and baptized at an early age, I was no stranger to exercising my faith. But keep in mind, I was a babe in Christ and as many of us, growing in discipleship.

However, this did not hinder me from seeking God in my difficult times. In fact, God and my *new* church family became my only support system that I trusted. Growing up in a southern Baptist church, I was taught the basics pertaining to doctrine and church protocol. Even though I was in the Sunshine choir, usher ministry and served as the Sunday school secretary at the small church rooted in the rural back roads of Clarksdale, Mississippi, I was not relationally or even spiritually connected to God. As a youth, everything I did while being a church member was out of tradition and formality. It remained this way up until my adolescent years. That is until one night I had an experience that truly was an epiphany of change.

One night, after I had moved off campus into my first apartment shared with others, I locked myself in my room and cried out to God like I had never done before. My television had been on one of the Christian network channels from surfing for some type of motivation, encouragement or hope. I had been halfway tuned in to the different televangelists who had either hosted their own broadcast or were guest on other shows. While kneeled and bent over with my forehead touching the floor, all of a sudden I heard this fiery Pentecostal male preacher's voice come through the airways of my room. It was as if God was speaking through him directly to me. As I continued to weep and cry out to God with a plethora of questions and complaints, the preacher would respond with answers as if we were in dialogue. I had never experienced anything like that before! Yes, as a child I was taught that we can talk to God and that He would answer, but I didn't expect Him to do it in that way. Oh, but my night got even more divine.

Still dismayed and nearly in shock about what was transpiring, it was awhile before I lifted my head up to look at my television. I didn't want the moment to end. I didn't know what was happening, but all I knew was that when I initially hit that floor, I had a void so deep and a pain so severe that it was going to take a miracle to help me. And I believe that is exactly what happened next.

"You, yes you, wailing on the floor right now. You are feeling broken, confused and you are hurting…God wants you to know that He loves you so much that He gave His only begotten Son just for you. He did not make the most ultimate sacrifice for you to remain in your condition….Your mind needs to be renewed and you need the Holy Ghost. If you believe and have confessed that Jesus is LORD and Savior, you shall receive the Holy Ghost and then you will have power! Did you hear what I just said? You shall have power!"

Yes, I remember all of that and then some about that night because I had never experienced anything like it before. I do realize that the various Christian denominations believe different doctrine and even as a student of theology, I will not argue that. But all I can testify to is my experience. I had come from a small church that never had 15 members on any given Sunday. The Dr. Watts and old time songs were all I knew. I didn't know anything about praise and worship or a Pentecostal experience. I had heard of the Holy Spirit, but didn't really see Him as a real entity with real power. After church on Sundays, I recall my Grandmother talking on the phone to her girlfriends about how it was an abomination for sister so and so to be speaking in tongues, which at the time I had no idea what that meant. And Lord knows I sure didn't do any dancing in church!

That night, I prayed to God like I had never done before. I praised and worshiped God like never before. I opened my Bible that I had been reading all of my life and I felt as if I was reading the Scriptures for the first time in my life. That night, the Word of God had been declared in my life like never before and I believed and received His Word. Although I had confessed Christ and had been baptized by my grandfather around the age of nine, every since that night, I have been telling everyone that I got saved at the age of 19. My faith became real to me that night and the enemy knew it too. But that night opened the door for me to enter into my final grief stage; accepting my brother's death. Which allowed me to eventually come to celebrating his life.

5 THE MASTER'S TOUCH

"Consider it pure joy, my brothers, whenever you face trials of many kinds, because you know that the testing of your faith develops perseverance." – James 1:2-3, NIV

The previous chapter ended on a relatively high note. I'm sure you will be able to relate to the transition in between. You have probably had your share of hard knockers in life that caused you to wobble as you fought to stand back up and face the rocks that life seems to constantly throw at you, rather than dodge them. You know that point you reach in life where you feel as though your faith has been tried and not only have you passed a mountain of tests, but have done so with excelling scores. And even those that you have failed gained you bragging rights because of the manner in which you applied what you learned from them. *So what happened on the other side of my victory?*

Was I really victorious in my circumstances? This is the doubt that the enemy tried to imprint in my mind. He constantly tried to plant untruths every opportunity he found me in a vulnerable state. I often remind myself and others that the enemy is patient and strategic. Again, we must remember that his plan has never changed: "The thief comes only to steal and kill and destroy" (John 10:10, NIV). Therefore, if we do not hold on to God's truths as soon as we learn of them, we will easily waver in our faith.

That experience I had in the bedroom of my apartment transpired during the early portion of the darkest years of my life. Undoubtedly, it was real. It was as though I had had a Damascus Road experience. Only during the time, I had no idea how my journey would be almost parallel to that of the apostle Paul. Immediately, I became an eye-witness for Christ. The 24 hours afterwards, I was compelled to tell those closest to me about what had happened. This continued for days, weeks, and months. It was as if a fire had been lit under my feet that just wouldn't allow me to be still or quiet.

The only person that could directly relate to my divine encounter and experience during that time was my college beau.

Reflecting from the aftermath, our story is filled with much irony. When we first met, I was the one with issues yet filled with *faith*. He was the seasonal churchgoer that his devout matriotic Christian grandmother kept on her prayer list. But because the prayers of the righteous availeth much (James 5:16), a transformation occurred in his life that became such a magnetic testimony. Initially, he started to have visions of himself being before crowds of people. Then he started being compelled to give up material things that he became convicted about. Before long he was regularly attending a local church in his area and was soon baptized physically and spiritually. And oh how he let his light shine and fire spread!

I was one of the first that he shared his experience with. Broadcast journalism was definitely the complimentary major for his calling. He relentlessly gave his eyewitness story to whomever would listen. Those that knew him from his hometown and on his college campus were really amazed. They knew him as an aspiring rapper, Casanova and party goer. So when they saw him become a consistent walking Gospel, whether or not they were among the many who were compelled to change their lives, they did respect the anointing that was so heavily upon him. And I, myself, could not help but reverence God's hand on his life. As the evangelist Gipsy Smith said, "There are five gospels of Jesus Christ – Matthew, Mark, Luke, John and you, the Christian. Many people will never read the first four."

God through my friend prompted the experience I had that night in my apartment. Ironically, the very person who I use to have arguments about not playing hardcore rap as we traveled to church was now the one witnessing to me about how I needed the baptism of the Holy Spirit. Sometimes it takes an unsaved person to save a religious person. I was reared Baptist and the church he had been attending and where he confessed Christ was Apostolic-Pentecostal. My religious traditions had me thinking that he was now a part of a cult. Never had I witnessed people speaking in tongues, shouting and dancing in the manner in which they did at his church and being *slain in the Spirit*. It was only until I had my own experiences that I knew theirs were authentic. But they didn't occur right away.

As excited as I was for my friend to know God in this new found way that he did, I was apprehensive about what was going on in his life. I had never witnessed any proclaimed Christian actually change as he had done. He really tried to apply and live out the Word of God. His faith had become so strong that without doubt he believed he could heal the sick. He didn't care who criticized him or did not believe him when it came to theological approaches. He stood firm on God's Word based upon his current interpretation and he constantly prayed for revelation. The rap music he use to tote was replaced by his new Bible that looked 10 years old in a matter of six months.

Why have I taken the time to tell you his story? For one, it is wrapped into mine. But also to paint a picture that most Believers can relate to: the first real encounter with Jesus and how the Holy Spirit really made a change in the carnal mind that became vivid in the natural body. For some, it has been forgotten. For many, life has caused you to repress it due to dreadful disappointments and unbelievable unpleasant situations. For all of us, the enemy has tirelessly worked hard to make us forget and even distrust the supernatural encounter that we had. The enemy knows that once we are turned right side up towards the light and away from darkness that his army just decreased in numbers. But when we as Christians are also constant in our faith, we will find ourselves winning more battles on the side of victory that we are already on.

My friend was the first non-relative that I expressed all of my challenging and negative experiences with. I shared things with him that I didn't even share with my family. He knew just about every shameful incident that I had experienced and yet always encouraged me. The difference was that after he got saved he believed that Jesus Christ was the answer to my breakthrough and healing. He continuously prayed for me and with me in a nonjudgmental way. Because he now had a relationship with God and saw how his old life did not parallel to his new one, he wanted everyone to have the opportunity to have this intimate relationship and not a religion. And a relationship was what I developed with God for myself and it was nothing short of amazing. Faith had manifested in my life.

It was a wonderful experience to be ministering together. There we were; two adolescents with past baggage that was endlessly trying to impede upon our present, boldly proclaiming the Good News, the Gospel of Jesus Christ. We attended mid-week services hosted by the Campus Crusade. We started campus Bible study ministries and ventured out to other colleges to host forums. We witnessed other people get saved or have breakthroughs. Despite the ridicule that we received from our family and friends, it was worth the true ministry that we were witnessing. God was definitely using us in an extraordinary way. And the enemy knew it. Little did we know that we were about to learn the context of Romans 8:28, "And we know that God causes everything to work together for the good of those who love God and are called according to his purpose for them."

A few months after we had our supernatural encounters, we had a natural event that altered our lives. One evening we were traveling from my aunt's wedding in Clarksdale, headed back to Oxford I had to be at work for the third shift that night at an answering service and we were already pressed for time. Under the assumption that I would have time to go to my apartment and change clothes, I still had on my maid of honor's fuchsia colored dress. We left my Grandmother's house in my 95' white Ford Escort destination Highway 6 East. It was in the month of May and the southern summer heat had already begun to fester. Midway to Marks, Mississippi, I pulled over to allow my friend to drive due to my fatigue. I figured I could get a nap in before having to work my scheduled eight hours of the third shift. Unknowingly to me, he was also exhausted from the long day; however, chivalry would not permit him to decline to drive. A few miles short of reaching Batesville, we collided head on with a pickup truck that had a horse trailer latched to it, which bolted a loose causing it to slam smack into the passenger side of my car.

I didn't know how long I had been asleep before the accident occurred. Upon impact, my friend had to swiftly pull me towards him in order to refrain me from being ejected from the car. Waking up to severe pain, it took me a minute before realizing a tragedy had just occurred. Thankfully, the adults and children in the other vehicle were all unharmed. My friend didn't have any major physical wounds either. But it was the sight of my condition that caused his emotional and even spiritual scars that he later shared with me.

Stretched out on the side of that Mississippi Delta highway in my friend's arms that night seemed like the longest wait for emergency assistance. My right foot was twisted inward and above it were peeled skin on my leg with blood flowing down from the cuts caused by shattered glass. My flat, petite stomach had inflated so that by the time the paramedics did arrive they thought I was three months to four months pregnant. In the time it took for the ambulance to transport me to the Batesville hospital, air lift me to the Elvis Presley Trauma Center, also known as the Med, in Memphis the release of internal fluids had caused me to appear to be in my third trimester.

The complicated surgery lasted several hours. It would be months later until I would realize how in depth my injuries were and just how God had blessed me to be alive. During the time, I didn't quite feel blessed. In addition to waking up to my family and friends; including the one who had experienced the traumatic experience with me, I woke up to a different me. There was a tube in my mouth that extended down my throat that hindered me from talking. There was the expected IV in my arm to allow the insertion of fluids and medications. What was unexpected was the feeding tube and catheter that had been inserted. My right foot and leg were covered in a hard cast. And as irritating as it was it did not compare to the soft cast that completely covered my abdomen. Underneath were the severity of my injuries. It was so bad that it took me two months later, when I was initially released from the hospital to even be able to look at my stomach.

A large tight band was placed on my stomach to help the skin that had been deeply cut from surgery to properly heal. There was a deep wound that was about two to three inches wide that started from the tip of my abdomen all the way down to about two inches below my navel. The reason for the lengthy surgery was because my pancreas had been punctured, my stomach had been torn and and my intestine had been ripped. I had been given what most people request as a weight loss procedure called gastric bypass. Therefore, one of the differences that soon came was with my weight. I went from wearing a 9-10 pants size to a two. And as I gradually learned, my mind had been affected by memory loss.

All of this definitely took some adjusting to. Laid up in that hospital room for months not being able to move or take care of my everyday hygiene on my own became depressing for me, becoming a part of my seven year battle with major depression. I felt as though the enemy was dancing on my new joy and what had seemed like my victory. But in the midst of it all, was a familiar voice that wouldn't allow me to give up.

6 WALKING IN FAITH

Depression: (major depressive disorder or clinical depression) "is a common but serious mood disorder. It causes severe symptoms that affect how you feel, think, and handle daily activities, such as sleeping, eating, or working. Symptoms are present for at least two weeks".[vi]

Perception and deception are powerful tools that feeds the mind. If your perspective is not rooted in positivity and the promises of God, then you will easily become deceived and manipulated by the words and works of the enemy. Joyce Meyer penned it best, there is a "Battlefield of the mind….and the mind is the battlefield" (2011).[vii]

Perhaps you too have found yourself experiencing a devastating trauma, one that has left you emotionally and mentally scarred right when you thought God was moving in an extraordinary way in your life. Then when disaster strikes, you are tranquilized by your perception of the tragedy rather than the reality of God's truth. As I did, you find yourself having a Job moment and start questioning God rather than speak bold declarations to the enemy. *Isn't it a wonder how he always feels so in charge of our lives?*

The Reality of Depression

Within the church, we come in contact with hurting people the most, yet, we paralyze ourselves and others from getting real help. Is it intentional? Not necessarily. Often times it is done out of ignorance. Other times it is done out of fear. We tend to fear what we don't understand and instead of stepping out of our comfort zone to educate ourselves about it, we ignore the reality of the emotions crying out right before us, as well as, within ourselves. When a mood disorder such as depression has taken root, it can be difficult to extract. And when other cavities or traumas occur simultaneously, it can cause even further decay. If you have ever had a toothache, then you can relate to my analogy.

Depression is a universal illness by which millions

can relate. And in order for everyone to gain a better understanding about the reality of depression it is relevant to be aware of the stigmas associated with mental illnesses; specifically depression, the types of depression and the causes of depression.

The Stigma

Depression is a real illness. It is a mental illness that affects not only the mind, but one's emotional and physical state. A person who is affected by depression cannot just "snap out" of it. There are many other stigmas associated with depression that hinders many from receiving help. Although mental health advocates have made significant progress in eradicating the stigma associated with just the term "mental illness" alone, there are still many communities that shy away from needed discussions and unfortunately, are even judgmental about the dialogue that occurs and critical of those that are affected by a mental illness.

1. *Social stigma.* Social stigma is a set of negative and often unfair beliefs that a society or group of people have about something.[viii] We have all probably been guilty of having a preconceived notion about something that was new to us.

Recall the first time you were introduced to the coupled words, mental illness or mental disorder. What were your first thoughts? I will go ahead and state what you are thinking and probably feeling guilty about thinking right now: That's associated with 'crazy' people or 'nut cases'. It's okay to confess this. Culturally, this has been our way of associating those dealing with depression or a mental disorder. We have placed them all in one basket without understanding the how and why. We automatically view them as being different and set a part from ourselves and end up labeling them in our workplaces, churches and homes.

2. *Self-stigma.* Self-stigma also known as perceived stigma, "occurs when people internalize these public attitudes and suffer numerous negative consequences as a result"[ix] Therefore, social and self-stigmas are related to one another. Those affected by depression frequently deal with the barrier of self-stigma because of how depression is negatively discussed or perceived within their communities or social environments.

Now, let us apply these stigmas specifically within the church. Many people of faith experience acute or chronic depression. As a matter of fact, most people are depressed even after attending their weekly worship services. Does this mean that the pastor or minister did not do his or her job in preaching an empowering and evangelical message? No. As someone who faithfully attended weekly church services as a layperson while experiencing depression, I can shed light on this answer.

During the active periods of my chronic depression, I still believed in God and His provision for my life; even though, I did not understand why I felt as low as I did. Despite the fact that my Saturday nights were mostly filled with constant wailing, continuous crying and desperate pleas for help, it was the hope that God would hear my cries, deliver me from my depression and heal my broken spirit (ref. Psalm 34:17-18) that allowed me to push my way to church on Sundays. I would force myself to participate in praise and worship and this was when I felt safe and comforted. I would be empowered by a sermon that provoked me to respond to an altar call. This is mostly where the ball would drop.

Prayer is a powerful weapon that we as Christian

believers have. James tells us that "the prayer offered in faith will make the sick person well; the Lord will raise him up. If he has sinned, he will be forgiven. Therefore confess your sins to each other and pray for each other so that you may be healed. The prayer of a righteous man is powerful and effective" (5:15-16).

If an intercessor, one praying for another or standing in the gap for someone, is not properly trained in the laws or principles of prayer, he or she is just speaking words in the air. The brave times that I would take the walk down the aisle and request prayer for my depression and even suicidal thoughts, I would either initially receive an expression that implied: *Christians don't get depressed* or *how dare you even speak of having such thoughts*. The intercessor would proceed to speak the words in prayer and once finished praying, would reiterate to me how I was just being used by satan. And although in a way this was true, because the enemy does work to attack our minds. But this was not the proper response to give to someone who had just made such a confession. Many ministers and intercessors are limited by their knowledge of depression and other disorders; therefore, hindering the effectiveness of their prayers and helping those they minister to.

Causes of Depression

Do you recall the Bible encounter when Jesus healed the man born blind and the naysayers wanted to find fault in the man and his parents? Well, in the ninth chapter of John, Jesus responded, "Neither this man nor his parents sinned...but this happened so that the work of God might be displayed in his life" (v. 3). Whereas sin can be an enabler for depression, it is not solely an absolute cause. And no, one does not have to be born with a disability in order to be affected by a mental illness.

1. *Stress.* Every day we encounter possible stressors. While there is good and bad stress, an unmanageable imbalance of it can cause us to become overwhelmed and lose our ability to properly function on a daily basis. This is why stress management is essential to our health.

2. *Death or a Loss.* Death is apart of the cycle of life. Although it is a normal event, sometimes it occurs in a natural or 'abnormal' way that results in a tragic loss. Regardless of how someone dies there is still the process of grieving that takes place. Not only do we mourn those we love. We also grieve over losing material things or even intangible things such as a job

or time we consider wasted or lost.

3. *Genetics.* Depression can be hereditary. Just as there are other illnesses and disorders that are passed through genes, so can depression and other mental illnesses be hereditary. Chemical imbalances affecting the brain also is a contributing factor for depression.

4. *Trauma.* Life changing events such as physical, emotional or sexual abuse, accidents and severe illnesses can trigger depression. My experience from the car accident traumatized me in a new way. It took years for my body to fully recover. And even then, I had to deal with physical side effects. In addition, it stimulated familiar emotional and mental side effects.

There are other additional causes of depression, but for the purposes of this book I have chosen to narrow the list. However, I do want to mention that substance abuse is also a cause stimulating depression. It's known as a dual diagnosis disorder, "a term for when someone experiences a mental illness and a substance abuse problem simultaneously".[x] This entails individuals that have an alcohol or drug addiction. Those affected by a dual diagnosis may be suffering from depression and choose to drink alcohol or partake in legal or illegal drugs as a way to deal with their problem. On the other hand, some substance abusers become depressed due to the side effects.

Another cause of depression that is relevant to mention is a term called *faulty thinking*. Faulty thinking consists of our incorrect thoughts about ourselves; untruths. Dr. Chris Thurman describes this way of thinking as "self-talk dictates our moods, our reactions, and even our maturity level in Christ." Our thoughts are powerful. What we think about ourselves is manifested in our mood, actions and relationships. As the Bible declares, "For as he thinketh in his heart, so is he" (Proverbs 23:7).

7 LEADING WHILE BLEEDING

"But he said to me, 'My grace is sufficient for you, for my power is made perfect in weakness'. Therefore I will boast all the more gladly about my weaknesses, so that Christ's power may rest on me. That is why, for Christ's sake, I delight in weaknesses, in insults, in hardships, in persecutions, in difficulties. For when I am weak, then I am strong. " – 2 Corinthians 12:9-10, NIV

Believe it or not, but every leader is human. This is true in the secular and spiritual realms. But leaders are more often perceived to be superman or woman and most criticized in the faith-based arena. One of the oldest clichés or proverbs is "never say never" or "never say what you wouldn't do". When you are on the opposite end of the spectrum, it is easy to declare what you would do in a certain polar position or situation. But it is only until you are faced with the challenge of moving to the family of blues or walking in someone else's shoes that you find yourself wanting to retract your bold statement.

Despite how God has declared that He has a plan for all of our lives, we do find ourselves quite often wondering *what is our purpose?* Quiet as it is kept many of us, even spiritual leaders, find ourselves wondering *if there is any point at all in discovering what that purpose is?* I have definitely been there. Many Christians have experienced seasons or intermissions in life when life itself does not seem worth living. It is one thing to deal with crises during our childhood, adolescent and baby Christian stages of life, but there is an expected tolerance when faced with such challenges as seasoned Saints. Because we have individually set such a high standard of expectation we nearly make it impossible for others and ourselves to receive or reach out for help.

In a way, ministers are like medical doctors when it comes to helping hurting people while sometimes hurting or suffering themselves. It would be deemed unprofessional, unethical or even insensitive for a doctor to vent to his bleeding patient that was rushed into the emergency room after being ejected from a vehicle, despite the fact that the surgeon himself is suffering severe stomach pain and is over due for a much needed surgery. In a similar manner, a minister normally doesn't share his hurts or thorns with an afflicted church member. Those intimate details are usually entrusted to a mentor, colleague or co-laborer in the ministry. But here is the downside; leaders don't even reveal everything to their confidants or those who can relate to their suffering because of the fear of being judged or labeled incompetent. I have been on the receiving end of such criticism.

So far, I have shared a couple of intimate details regarding experiences in my life. Hopefully, you have not had to experience any of them. Unfortunately, too many of you have had very similar occurrences or know acquaintances that have. After having gone through devastating events in your life and finding yourself on the side of victory, life reminds you that there are many more battles. These battles can really mess with your mind. It isn't necessarily the intensity of the battlefields, rather the timing in which they arrive. It is one thing to have to fight in private, but another thing to have to fight your battles on public display and with your *enemies* watching and waiting for your defeat.

I have already revealed the darkest hour of my life; the aftermath of my brother's suicide. But even after having *survived* that place of desperation and desolation, to land in a desert storm was one of the loneliest and lost periods that I have experienced. It was a state where I found myself leading while bleeding. I was leading in the sense that I had started to become known as the poster child of hope for those dealing with depression, suicidal thoughts or survivors of suicide. I was leading in the sense that I had been called into the Gospel ministry, ordained in ministry, serving as an associate pastor and found myself once again bleeding the darkness of a mental disorder.

I do not know the exact day that initiated what was labeled my nervous breakdown. I do not know the exact event or incident that triggered what appeared to be my downfall. What I do vividly recall is the exact moment when I received the revelation that I had deviated off the highway called my life. It was one Sunday during late spring when I was about to minister and found myself standing out on the visiting church's parking lot having a conversation with God; although, it was not an audible or verbal dialogue. That moment of epiphany was driven by a series of what I considered spiritual calamities. I felt paralyzed by the magnitude of spiritual abuse that seem to be growing rapidly throughout congregations. I was numbed by the guilt of my rebellious response of intentionally making my ministry gifts inactive. This, plus the normal day-to-day sinner's conviction had me tremendously grieved in spirit by the preconceived notion that I had greatly disappointed God.

Standing in the anguish of failure with the pressing assignment to communicate the Gospel behind me, while my own communication with God was distorted was such a heavy weight to bare. This, plus everything that was going on in my life made me feel as though I was suffocating in agony. I must have appeared to have it all together because everyone was using me as a part of their support system, seeking me for counsel and requesting consultations for various matters. I was constantly pouring out, but nothing was being replenished. Eventually, I suffered the consequence that almost ended my life.

Throughout every traumatic and tragic event that caused me to be affected by a mental disorder, any mishandling of my health care never came from professionals. That was until this particular depressive episode that caused me to be detained for nearly a month in a facility that was not a hospital. You see, there are other entities that stigmatize and cause barriers to treating those with mental illnesses. Unfortunately, there are governing bodies that are also uneducated about issues pertaining to mental health care; therefore, causing their states not to be updated with relevant laws, policies and services. As a result, there are too many emergency room cases that involve suicidal attempts where trauma patients are discharged to institutions meant to punish criminals. Can you imagine being in an accident that caused you severe physical injuries prompting paramedics to rush you to the ER for help and instead of the medical team treating your injuries they treat you like a criminal? This was not only my case, but as I terribly had to learn, this was the treatment plan for many minor and even severe mental health cases.

Why or How? Is probably what you have just asked yourself. Well, not only did I ask myself those questions, but respectively I asked God too. Our dialogue, especially from my end, did not consist of short rebuttals. I sincerely wanted God to explain to me how He could have called me out of darkness only to be thrown into a tunnel. I wanted to know how He could have called me out of a box only to be pitched into a ditch? How could He have called and chosen me to teach and preach the Gospel of Good News only to make me the sidebar conversation of mere *gossip*?

Having already experienced what it felt like to be a spectacle as a lay person seeking the church for help, as a minister, I faced the harsh reality of having friends in the ministry and spiritual leaders to ostracize me while experiencing another episode of major depressive disorder. It was one thing to deal with the disappointment of not being able to confide and receive comfort from those that had declared to be concerned about my spiritual walk and claimed to be my friend, but to have the same people who once called me in the middle of the night for prayer and spiritual counsel now treat me like a castaway, felt like a jagged edge being ripped from my side.

Fortunately, I can say that I was and am blessed to have a core group a part of my support system that have never intentionally judged me. Even if they did not understand what I was going through emotionally, they were genuine enough to offer raw support without any stigma attached. And when you have been told by a friend that their doors are always open to you and the one night they have to uphold their word they choose to let you sleep inside your car, you can really appreciate the friendship from those who actively, privately and publicly show it.

But what about the church? Unfortunately, during that time I was under the leadership of a pastor who did not understand mental health issues or disorders and rather than seek education or resources to help he chose to scandalize my name by placing a label on me among the ministerial staff and congregation. Can you imagine how painful it was to hear conversations attacking your moments of weaknesses by the one who is suppose to be constantly praying for you, the one who weekly calls on you to teach Bible study and to fill in to preach Sunday morning worship service? Now, you might be wondering what was my response to this spiritual abuse and betrayal? And the answer is advocacy.

I resorted to what had become natural and even therapeutic for me; advocating for mental health.

Honestly, I did not want to give this initial response. Within myself, I had to deal with the ugly feelings of bitterness that tried to override my longing for inner and external peace. But I didn't have the energy or time to linger long in a place of trying to explain to allegedly seasoned and mature Christians the connection between spiritual captivity and mental illness, which I will delve further into in the next chapter. But because I had a good support system that included authentic prayer warriors, friends whose professional background allowed them to be able to give sound advice and most importantly my faith in the promises of God, I was able to rise above the low blows.

Rather than engage in an unhealthy confrontation among spiritual leadership, I chose to advocate more through the vehicle of education within the church and local community. I knew this response would be effective in the long run, but I didn't know the depth of its immediate results. While church leadership was busy manifesting the fear of what they didn't understand through toxic conversations, the members of the congregation were secretly calling me on the phone, requesting meetings with me or stopping me on the church parking lot after giving no response to the pastor's altar call, to confide in me about their personal struggles or someone in their family.

Depression had hit their families and some of their teenagers had expressed thoughts of suicide. But they were too ashamed to seek help from their pastor who in most cases they had known longer than they knew me. They were desperate for help and they felt comfortable reaching out to some one who could not only relate to them, but who would not judge or condemn them for verbalizing their real emotions or accuse them of not having enough faith. And as you can probably perceive, seeking professional help outside of the church was not an option they were receptive to or at least not ready to openly admit they were. The reality is that a great number of people turn to the church in their desperate times whether they are an avid believer or not. But the church is not always in a position of reality to help them.

According to the New York Times, "Members of the clergy now suffer from obesity, hypertension and depression at rates higher than most Americans. In the last decade, their use of antidepressants has risen, while their life expectancy has fallen. Many would change jobs if they could" (Aug. 1, 2010). Research and clinical reports show that many clergy are affected by mental disorders. This revelation is not new. However, the reported cases have increased throughout the years. This further reveals that the weight of trying to carry the burdens of the congregation simultaneously with personal problems have been heavy enough to cause pastors to seek resources outside of their spiritual realm for help. Of course this is a good thing. It signifies strength. Strength that church members need to see among their spiritual leaders that will signal it is okay to acknowledge when you need help and receive that help from an outside resource. Although the church has made some progress toward helping leaders who are bleeding out anxiety, burnout, depression, grief and other emotional disorders, there is a particular segment of the faith-based community that is still struggling to embrace these outside resources; the Black church. This draws me back to my story.

In addition to laity reaching out to me for help, ministers also started confiding in me about their struggles with depression. And even though I would not want anyone to experience the emptiness and loneliness that I had, it was reassuring to know that I could provide support to colleagues because I could simply relate to them. I was very familiar with the distant look of despair that was fixated in their eyes and the struggle of reluctance delivered in their voices. Even so, gaining this confidence did not occur overnight. Regrettably, in many instances it took tragedies among clergy on the national and even local level for ministers to yield themselves to vulnerability and scrutiny.

News of clergy losing their lives to suicide started to kindle through media outlets forcing churches to engage in unwanted conversations. Although it was much needed dialogue, in many cases it was not healthy conversation; especially within the Black church and community. Pastors did not know how to facilitate dialogue on such a sensitive subject. They themselves did not understand the tragedy of a life lost to suicide. Many were torn over determining their personal stand. For many it was a matter of morality, ethics, doctrine or all three. Not only did they have to try and explain what seemed to be the unexplainable to their own congregations, but some had to muster the strength to comfort and reinforce hope to the members of those pastors who were the victims of suicide. How does one explain to a member that their spiritual leader who weekly encouraged them not to give up on God decided to end his own life?

Providing pastoral counseling to these members was quite challenging for spiritual leaders. In the midst of these tragedies, pastors had to acknowledge that not only do they have common struggles as other Christians, but that they too were not exempt from being affected by mental disorders. As tragic as it was to learn of ministers attempting or successfully executing an act of suicide, it set off a panic alarm that could not be ignored. Church leaders started reaching out to me, other experts and organizations for help. Initially, it was mainly to assist with postvention. Despite this small step towards advocacy, in order to break real barriers, progress in the areas of prevention and intervention had to be made. This is a part of the ultimate goal.

8 THE SILENT KILLER

Suicide: "There is no single cause to suicide. It most often occurs when stressors exceed current coping abilities of someone suffering from a mental illness."[xi]

In chapter two I shared how silence is a barrier for those hurting to get help. When someone is hurting, the afflicted area of need is a major factor; however, it is not the most critical concern. Regardless if someone is in emotional, physical or mental pain they will not receive the help they need if no one is aware they are in need of assistance. For instance, if someone passed by a burning vehicle and saw a person trapped inside, the fact that the victim could not be heard would not prevent a by passer from trying to help them. But who pays attention to the warning signs of someone trapped inside a hopeless mind?

Silence Kills

Suicide is a silent killer and "It is the most preventable cause of death".[xii] Yet, so many lives are lost every year because of it. As described in the previous chapters, the illness does not discriminate based upon age, race, economic or social status. According to the American Foundation for Suicide Prevention, in 2014 suicide was the 10th leading cause of death in the United States, the highest rate was among the age group 85 and older, the second highest rate was in the age range 45-64, and it was the third leading cause of death among those between the age of 15-24. Despite how disturbing these statistics are, due to lack of reporting, they do not reflect absolute findings.

Stigma causes many cases to go unreported. Shame, guilt, and lack of knowledge causes family members of those loved ones who died by suicide from getting the help they need in order to live life beyond the tragic loss. This enables the cycle of the silent killer to continue. The cycle of silently living with suicidal thoughts must stop. The way to stop it is to give it a voice. When it is confessed, discussed and advocated this brings awareness and fosters an avenue for help. In case you are thinking it is the responsibility of those hurting to say they need help, then perhaps I have failed to describe and explain why it is not solely up to them and why in most cases, it can not be at all. Their silence doesn't mean that they don't want help. Stigma and the mental disorder itself tells them that help is not a present option.

Suicide, Youth and Adolescents

My brother, Marchello, is why I advocate strongly for teens. Because of my brother and my own personal experiences, I can empathize and relate to teenagers who are overwhelmed by anxiety, depression and even suicidal thoughts. During my speaking engagements at youth organizations, churches and schools, teens open up to me, a stranger, about their feelings and thoughts after I have shared my story. It is heart breaking to watch the tears roll down the cheeks of teenage girls and remember that same pain I had at their age. It is devastating to watch teenage boys breakdown among their peers because they had been holding their emotions hostage inside. When both of these genders and age groups are asked why haven't they told anyone what is going on with them, the general response is the same: *We don't talk about stuff like that in my family.*

We didn't talk about depression and suicide in my family either. This is probably one of the reasons why my 15-year-old brother didn't think he could reach out to anyone for help. This is primarily why I couldn't reach out to my family for help. And when I did, the fear that so many teens and adults have was manifested; being labeled and ostracized. As a matter of fact, after surviving one of my suicide attempts as an adolescent, instead of being comforted and loved on by my family, I was verbally and physically abused. In retrospect, I do not think the root reason was because they did not care, but because they feared what they did not understand. Nevertheless, this caused me to shut down and isolate myself even further. And it also caused me to gravitate to abusive and unhealthy relationships. When youth do not receive the proper help or response to tragedy or trauma, they end up seeking unhealthy solutions and become hurting adults with no resolve.

Another population that I advocate for are college students. Recall the statistics that revealed high suicide rates among the age group 15-24. College students fall within this range. Attending college can be very exciting for a first time college student who has been waiting 18 years to explore the world post high school and beyond the confinements of their parents. However, the long anticipated freedom also comes with challenges, obligations and responsibilities.

College students encounter new stressors. Peer pressure remains a factor as it did during high school, but on a different scale. There is the challenge of trying to balance academics with the extremes of a social life, the conflict of trying to please parents while pursuing personal goals and dealing with the pressure of any past problems or tragedies that are impeding in the present. As enthusiastic and social friendly college life can be it can also be an island or desert quick sand to an overwhelmed student. And with no immediate access to mom or dad, who is left to zoom into the life of a drifting or drowning adolescent?

My college saying on friendship was that, *If you befriend a person your freshman year and you manage to still be friends with that person after college, then you can probably consider that person a lifetime friend.* Many college students are blessed to gain friendships that they feel comfortable enough to confide in. At times this was definitely true for me. But when this truth does not hold to be factual for college students, parental involvement should be active. Parental engagement should not be a back up plan for support, but it should be the core of a college student's support system. Many parents believe that they have the type of relationship that their children feel as though they could tell them anything. Unfortunately, it is only until tragedy hits that they realize they were wrong.

Suicide and the Church

<u>The Faith Community</u>

Mental disorders affect people of faith from all denominational and religious backgrounds. Because I am a Christian believer, I have chosen to focus on this area of faith. I believe I have already proven that Christians are not exempt from experiencing mental health disorders whether or not it is acute or chronic. But even though the Bible is clear in stating this fact, I believe it is necessary to frequently reiterate that Christians are neither exempt from trials, temptations or tribulations. It is not non-believers who need convincing; rather, it is the confessed Christian. A large segment of the Christian community stigmatizes any phrase associated with the words *mental health*, *mental disorders* or *mental illnesses*.

Nine times out of ten you are a Christian believer;

therefore, I do not think you need further convincing that it is possible for a born again believer to have suicidal thoughts. Of course I am not suggesting that you personally have had such ponderings. But perhaps you know of someone who has discretely confided in you or heard of a particular incident at your church or within your community. Which ever the case, that person, that Christian did not all of a sudden arise with death on his or her mind or the boldness to act on a permanent decision.

At some point during a Christian's walk, he or she believes that God cares for them, that He wants to comfort them and that He wants to carry their heavy burdens. But somewhere in between receiving another disappointment, another rejection and being used, mistreated and hurt one too many times by others and even other Christians they reach a place that they never thought they would. Who would they share their darkness with? Who within the church would not criticize them for not having enough faith? Who in the church would offer another solution other than prayer? Is prayer effective and necessary for a suicidal Christian? Yes! But after prayer, then what? Even the Bible tells us in the book of James that "faith by itself, if it is not accompanied by action, is dead" (2:17, NIV).

The Black Community

When I first started advocating for mental health on social media several years ago, I created a page entitled "Breaking Mental Health Barriers in the Black Community". The page attracted diverse followers. As a result, I received modest criticism from a few individuals. They were not offensive, at least not to me because they were relevant questions and concerns that I used as teaching moments for my collective audience. Basically, they inquired why I signaled out a particular race when in fact everyone is impacted by mental illnesses in some manner? The fact that they posed this particular question confirmed two things: 1) They were advocates and therefore aware of the pressing need to help those affected and 2) They were apparently unaware of the stigma attached to certain populations that causes more of a barrier for them to receive help.

Creating this particular page definitely was not intended to suggest that other populations are not affected by mental illnesses. But it was formed to bring awareness that certain populations, particularly the black community are in desperate need of mental health services. Research indicates that other populations voluntarily receive more professional services for their mental health conditions. As a result this impacts the statistics on the number of African-Americans affected by mental illnesses. Because the black community is unlikely to seek professional support when dealing with a mental condition, there are many cases that go unreported. Why is this a fact?

Stigma. It goes back to the negative connotation associated with mental illness. The black community is no stranger to experiencing a high degree of stereotypes. But the mental health stereotype mostly comes from within. Throughout black history; slavery, Civil Rights and the now Black Lives Matter movement the African-American community has been known for its strength and high level of resilience. Therefore, to be viewed as not mentally strong is considered a sign of weakness. So who does the black community turn to for help or support?

The black church has been the backbone of support for the African-American community. It is the safe haven for those needing refuge, replenishing and restoring. It is the sacred place you go when you are hurting privately and even hurting while on public display. It is the place you go to because you have hope in your faith and your faith gives you hope that things will get better. African-Americans are most likely to consult with their pastor first before their doctor or another professional. Since the church is the primary source that the black community relies on and trusts, it should also be the vehicle to mental health advocacy.

9 KEEPING MY FAITH

"Now faith is the substance of things hoped for, the evidence of things not seen" (Hebrews 11:1, KJV).

How does anyone keep their faith while saving their mind? The same way they would keep their faith while encountering any trauma; by standing firm. Sounds too simple? Perhaps because you were expecting a more profound response. When you are going through terrifying moments that try to shake your faith, you have to remember that you are in a battle. What does a soldier do to prepare for warfare? He gets suited up with the right gear.

The Bible tells us in Ephesians to "Put on the full armor of God so that you can take your stand against the devil's schemes" (6:11, NIV). The devil does not grow tired or restless from his tricks. But he diligently works to wear us out. So we as Christian believers must stand strong on our faith. We have to stand when we are experiencing internal conflict and trust that God is going to deliver us out of our bondage. We have to stand even when others in the faith seem to be standing against us. What I first observed through my trials was that when I would experience low moments that would cause me to waver in my faith was when I paid more attention to the noise surrounding me. Every time that I would allow my mind to wonder off of Jesus; the Word, prayer time, praise and worship, I would feel myself sinking. It reminds me of the time when the apostle Peter was walking on water at Jesus' command and when he took his eyes off of Jesus, he started sinking (ref. Matthew 14:30). One thing that I do know is that flesh will fail, but faith does not.

When you find yourself feeling as though your faith is failing you, I challenge you to look within. God's Word never changes because He never changes. There is always more of Him to know, but we have to allow ourselves to draw closer to Him every day. In doing so, we gain wisdom, knowledge and direction. These three are imperative when dealing with traumatic experiences and even mental illnesses whether the disorder itself is a primary problem or a side effect. Faith should not be seen as a barrier to getting help with mental disorders. Especially when in actuality it is the terminology used that causes the barrier.

You see, within the church, we want to cling to the term spiritual captivity because it sounds spiritual and we can personally and publicly declare that as our issue when we don't really understand what it really entails. But mental illness is in the realm of spiritual captivity. And when dealing with it from the faith arena, it needs to be understood that you can counsel and cast out.

Do you recall the story of the demon-possessed man? One of the narratives can be found in the fifth chapter in the book of Mark. His story really capitulates how we as *church folks* handle people not just with mental issues, but any issue.

1) **We try to bind what we don't understand**. In verses three and four of this passage, the people had tried to physically chain the man who was labeled in our modern time as 'crazy'. But the man continuously broke the chains and isolated himself in a tomb. Obviously no one was able to spiritually comprehend what they were dealing with because they were providing the wrong

solution.

2) **We allow our ignorance about issues cause them to escalate.** The second part of verse four says that "No one was strong enough to subdue [tame] him." How was it permitted to allow this demon-possessed man's power to grow out of control to the point that the *church folks* could not handle him?

3) **We don't use our authority over demons or issues.** Jesus' presence alone brought this man out of his captivity. The demon-possessed man not only ran towards Jesus, but respected and acknowledged His authority by kneeling before Him. After Jesus identified and called out the man's issue, the man who had been bound and untamed by man was now delivered. Why didn't the man fear or reverence the authority in the people? I understand the semantics of this text concerning the audience. But sometimes we as church folks are not walking in our authority; therefore, the enemy does not fear us. If we are not walking in our authority we are unable to use our authority to speak and command the enemy.

4) **We don't accept deliverance.** After Jesus delivered the man that had been bound and repositioned

him back in his "right mind" (v. 15), the people rejected what they had witnessed instead of rejoicing. They even asked Jesus to leave their town!

Sometimes people don't want you delivered because they have become content with knowing you by your issue. Some people thrive off of what they consider to be the weaknesses of others because it some how makes them appear stronger. While secretly, they either don't want to admit they are not able to help you or because they are dealing with similar issues themselves. In my teaching ministry, I once used the Bible passage from Second Samuel to expound on this. It states that, "Now David had been told, 'Ahithophel is among the conspirators with Absalom.' So David prayed, 'O LORD, turn Ahithophel's counsel into foolishness" (15:31, NIV). You would need to read the entire chapter and book more thoroughly to gain a full understanding and appreciation of the text. But my personal commentary simply crosses the river this way: Do not worry about those who insist to speak against you. No matter how wise, influential or smart they appear. GOD knows how to make them an unreliable source!

Keeping your faith has nothing to do with church or

religion. Now I have grown past the notion that a particular denomination is the basis for salvation, healing or deliverance. However, I do realize, believe and know that being in a place of worship that allows you to get in a position for praise and worship makes a difference from one being held captive and set free. In other words, when I was at churches that acknowledged, embraced, and executed all areas of five-fold ministry it prepared, sanctified an atmosphere for a deliverance ministry. But before people can get to the point of deliverance, their issue has to be called out. Not called out in the sense that someone stands up in the pulpit and call them by their earthly names, but allowing the Spirit of God to call out the demonic stronghold within them (ref. Mark 5:8).

What does this mean for the church? If you are the member or visitor seeking help or solutions, this means that attending a live church is vitally important not only for your spiritual growth, but how you weather through carnal storms. What do I mean by a *live* church? One that is not dead. When you are faced with some of the darkest days of your life, you can not afford to be a part of a captive audience that serves as a parasite to your remaining joy. You need to be at a church that preaches and teaches the Word of God and not a watered down message or an emotionalized sermon. You need to be at a church that allows you to be free to cry out, sing and dance unto the Lord and not look at you funny when you do so. You need to be at a church that can connect to God through every level of prayer and not give you a rehearsed prayer every Sunday. When you feel as though you are barely hanging on to life, you need to be at a place that has the ability to spiritually and if need be physically resuscitate you. In order words, a dead church is the last place a suicidal person needs to be!

If you are a pastor or a ministry leader and serious about ministering to God's people, this means that you are responsible for fostering the atmosphere I just described. No, it is not you who makes it alive. But do not let it be you who contributes to its deadness. As a minister your role is to minister to the saved and the unsaved. It is to help the hopeless. It is to do the works of Christ that you have been given authority to do. You are responsible for operating in your gifts and under the anointing. People do not have the time for you to play around with demons. You can not be a lip-service minister with no power to rebuke or release. If you lack the wisdom to minister, ask God for help (ref. James 1:5). If you lack the knowledge of the Scriptures to minister, then enhance your studies (ref. 2 Timothy 2:15). If you lack understanding of life issues, then seek the resources you need to minister effectively (ref. Proverbs 4:7). When you find yourself leading while bleeding, be humble enough to take care of yourself (ref. 1 Corinthians 6:19-20).

We as believers are all a part of the Body of Christ. We all have roles. We all have obligations and responsibilities to one another. Faith works in our lives when we work it. There is no failure in having faith in God; His Son Jesus, His Holy Spirit or His written Word. All three of these entities are at work and always available. When we are weak, we must have a spiritual support system who can pray without ceasing, praise in spite of and prophesy the promises of God to us. But even when this relevant team is unavailable, we have to be able to encourage ourselves through those things that are truth. We have to declare the Word of God over our lives; our situations, our issues and our conditions.

Faith Declarations

God has promised me power when I am weak.

- Isaiah 40:29

God has promised me strength and peace.

-Psalm 29:11

I can call upon God to heal me.

-Psalm 30:2

God has promised to heal my broken heart.

-Psalm 147:3

God has the power to heal me from evil spirits and release me from bondage.

-Mark 5:2-5

I do not have to be held captive by my past.

-Romans 8:1

God has not given me a spirit to fear.

-2 Timothy 1:7

Even in this, God is giving me the ability to endure so that I might become stronger.

-Colossians 1:11

God has declared that I shall not die, but live.

-Psalm 118:17

God does not have a plan to harm me.

-Jeremiah 29:11

God wants me to prosper.

-Jeremiah 29:11

God wants me to reap joy.

-Psalm 126:5

God has declared me more than a conqueror.

-Romans 8:37

Continue to add more of God's promises to these declarations. Memorize them. Believe them. Walk in them. Then, you will see your faith made stronger.

10 SAVING MY MIND

"Mental Health is defined as a state of well-being in which every individual realizes his or her own potential, can cope with the normal stresses of life, can work productively and fruitfully, and is able to make a contribution to her or his community."[xiii]

How do you save your mind while keeping your faith? I am not a psychologist or psychiatrist, but I am an expert witness to the facts of my own life. Keeping my faith has not just been about simultaneously saving my mind, but also keeping my faith through every day challenges and seasonal storms. However, it has been my mind, winning the fight for my sanity, that has exercised my faith the most. I know that I am not the only one who has struggled with keeping a healthy mind. The mind is what the enemy seeks to destroy. This is why it is critical that our minds are renewed (ref. Romans 12:2) and that we be clothed in the mind of Christ (ref. Philippians 2:5). Whereas, there is a spiritual, faith-based approach to maintaining a healthy mind it also includes other relevant elements.

The Approach to Saving the Mind

Hopefully, because I have shared intimate details about my life it will allow you to be further open to my transparency. One of the barriers that I faced when reaching out for help with family, friends and church members about my depression was having been made feel like I was less than human and incompetent to even have a say so about my own wellness. Due to confidential conversations, I know that others have also encountered the same experience. Yes, there are some mental illnesses that are so severe that causes a person not to be able to make any sound decisions about his or her life. But remember, you can not place all mental health cases in the same category.

<u>Health Care Includes the Mind</u>

If you were to learn during a routine wellness visit with your primary health care physician that you have high blood pressure, diabetes or even cancer, what would be your response? Depending upon which diagnosis, your natural reaction might be of shock. But once you get passed this stage you want to know your options. Therefore, you engage in an informative discussion with your doctor about your treatment plan and together you decide your course of action. Throughout the process, your doctor will ask you if the treatment plan seems to be working or if you are having any side effects to any medications that might be further affecting your health or your daily activities. Your physician, if an ethical one, will not treat you like a rat project or a guinea pig.

<u>Mental Health Care Includes the Person Affected</u>

When people consult with a doctor about a physical illness or diagnosis, they are given options and made to feel a part of the treatment plan. This is the same way that a mother dealing with postpartum depression, a grieving widow and even an over stressed adolescent should be treated. They should not be viewed as too incompetent to make a decision about their medical care or judged for being honest about their current mental state. Preventing someone affected by a mental disorder such as anxiety, bipolar or mild depression to voice their real feelings or emotions causes them to suffer silently, which does not prevent their condition from progressing to a severe stage. Then when they have arrived at a point where they can not make sound decisions social stigma has become a barrier for intervention. This definitely does not contribute to the goal of producing an outcome of no more lives lost. Rather someone is born with a mental illness or developed one during life, they can be at risk for suicide. It doesn't matter how someone became mentally ill. The ultimate goal for all is still the same; saving the life.

A Support System is Vital to Mental Health

The barrier of social stigma for those affected by a mental health disorder has to be removed when it comes to accessing mental health services. Once removed it will hinder self-stigma from interfering with those affected to reach out for support. A good support system is crucial to helping someone with an acute and definitely chronic mental illness. This support is comprised of those that the person in need trusts; therefore, it is hand picked by the person dealing with the mental illness.

People normally select their primary support system from three categories; family, friends and faith believers.

These are often the least people educated about their mental conditions and are the most criticizing. The most informed and those that have the ability to help the person; the physicians, counselors, social workers, mental health agencies and advocacy centers are usually chosen as secondary or not at all. So now, you can identify where the ball drops. And if it is going to keep the game of *life* going, it has to be picked up by the right players. Because the ball is not going to be thrown to the most popular or skilled, but the one who the guard trusts and relies on the most.

Enabling a Support System

What makes a great team is very similar to what it takes to make a great support system. A player knows his team mates; their strengths, their roles and their motives. He doesn't focus on their weaknesses while the game is going on because when he is holding the ball, he is the weakest link. All the players on the opposing team are coming after him. Everyone on his team is now stronger than he is. It is this strength that will allow them to operate effectively in their roles. They are motivated to play their roles because they all have a unified motive; to win the game.

When you are in the fight for saving your mind due to different life traumas or tragedies, you need people on your team who care if you win. One of the hardest blows I have faced during my chronic depressive episodes is to learn that people I have trusted; therefore, positioned on my support team really didn't care if I survived at all. They were only on my 'team' to be known as the VIP player regardless if it cost them a teammate.

If someone entrusts you to be a part of their support system, offer authentic support. If for what ever reason you can not, do not play around with their lives. Being genuinely supportive does not mean you have to be their savior or superhero. It means that you have a strength that they need to get them over the hurdle. That strength could be that of an encourager or prayer warrior. You could be selected because you are the one they can trust to 'tell it like it is' when they need the hard truth. You could be chosen because of your role in the community that links you to resources. They know it is a possibility that they might escalate to a point where they need professional help and in the event they do not have the strength to go themselves, they have a liaison and confidant in you.

The Church as the Primary Resource

I found it very intriguing to learn that "the pioneer and founder of clinical pastoral education (CPE), Anton Boisen, lived his entire live battling schizophrenia".[xiv] He obviously was in tuned about the connection between the church and mental health care. Since the church is the first place that Christians come to when they have problems and where even nonbelievers seek refuge, it makes sense for it to be equipped to effectively triage the needs of those they serve. This means that the pastoral or ministerial staff, ministry leaders, trustees and laity should work together to ensure that the church is ready to help those that come to them with some of the issues that I have discussed throughout this book.

Grief

The church is the main place that is connected to those grieving. It is the church that helps families go through the process of planning their loved ones memorial and burial services. This process is a journey within itself. Many words are declared at eulogies; words of comfort are given, promises are made to follow up and reminders are given declaring how much our brothers and sisters in Christ mean to us. Unfortunately, in too many cases they are empty words. They aren't meant to be. It is just that we have become so comfortable with going through the process of planning and protocol that we do not really dissect what the words mean to those on the receiving end. It is only until it is our time to grieve that we really appreciate the value of these traditional sayings.

Grief does not end after we leave the grave site. It is there that it truly begins. Not only do we want to ensure that our local church family is at fellowship the following Sunday, but we want to check on their emotional and spiritual needs. You might be thinking that this is the role of the pastor or ministerial team. And it is. It is also the responsibility of the entire church.

Here are a few brainstorming questions to consider with your soul care team or ministry group when ministering to church members dealing with grief:

1. **Other than the pastor, is there someone designated to follow up with members who have experienced the death of a loved one?** Due to the size variations of churches, the demands also varies. Even in a church small enough for the pastor to handle all the soul care needs, it should not be expected or demanded of

him or her. This will cause burnout and cause many members to fall through the crack.

2. **Is there an assessment conducted on the family?** When initial meetings with families occur, it is only to handle the service arrangements. There should also be a post-meeting with the immediate family to assess their needs. When death occurs, it causes a change in family dynamics. There might be a widow woman who is now left to handle all the financial affairs for her family. There might be a widow man who is now left to raise his children. If the deceased loved one was a child, are there any siblings that need help maneuvering through the grief process?

3. **Was the death expected or did it occur in a tragic way?** No death is a greater loss than the other. As previously mentioned, when a loved one has been ill it can allow the news to be received differently because family members would have had time to prepare themselves emotionally. Either way, grief still has to run its course. But what about the type of grief that I experienced with my brother? Given my own

experience and those that I have ministered and counseled, suicide is the most difficult grief to process. Mainly because beginning the process can be very hard and confusing. It ultimately leaves you with no one to blame and the person you want to vent at is no longer here. After blaming self, it can cause you to blame God. It can cause you to want to be distant from God and near Him at the same time. How does the church help someone grieving in this manner? Yes, prayer. But again, after prayer, then what? God has promised to help those brokenhearted and crushed in spirit. And yes, God can do a miraculous solo act. But He created us for relationships. He works through people. Is your church prepared to help those grieving from a death by suicide? Does your church have resources available for those grieving in this manner?

Sexual Abuse

Recall the young woman I mentioned in chapter two that came to the church's Bible study for help after she had been assaulted. There are countless number of individuals who have walked in her same shoes. Regrettably, too many of them never voice their own plea for help. As previously outlined, there are stages that must occur in order for victims of sexual abuse to receive help. Now, the church may not be oblivious to all of the stages because the situation simply has not been revealed to them. But when the church has received knowledge that a member of the congregation has been sexually abused it should actively be involved in the Getting Help stage. It does not matter whether or not the information was revealed at the altar through prayer, during a pastoral counseling session, or at a small group meeting. It does not matter whether the act took place outside or within the church. Here are a few questions to consider:

1. **Does the church have anyone trained to help victims of sexual abuse?** A person who has been sexually assaulted needs the spiritual and emotional support from their trusted church family. But depending upon the status of the abuse; whether or not it is currently ongoing or a past occurrence, they will also need help connecting to professional resources. The church should have a person or ministry assigned for this

role. It doesn't necessarily have to be a designated staff person, but it could be a volunteer church member who already works in this area of expertise.

2. **Does the church offer training or informational sessions to its leaders and entire congregation?** Most times it is the general congregation who learns of cases involving sexual abuse because the victim has confided in them. In which case, they either go directly to the pastor or a member of church leadership for help or accompany the victim. Leadership needs to receive training on how to handle such referrals and laity needs to be informed on who to contact within the church for help. If the victim is a child, leadership members need to know their roles and responsibilities.

Depression

Statistics indicate that there are more people dealing with forms of depression than any other mental disorder or trauma I have discussed. The fact that depression can be a side effect to crisis situations, as well as, the main crisis is a contributing benefactor. Although it is not the church's role to serve as a clinical facility per se, but because the church is connected to so many people dealing with depression it is obligated to assist its congregants in receiving help. Here are ways to do so:

1. **Trained Ministers.** Ministers will either be the first to receive notice of church members dealing with depression and the ones designated to offer pastoral counseling. Ongoing training is needed to equip them in doing so. This will allow them to know when outside referrals need to be made and help keep acute depression referrals from escalating.

2. **Healthy Ministry.** Many churches have embraced advocating for healthier lifestyles and have created health ministries. A great deal of them have designated health ambassadors who are trained to advocate, educate and even in some cases provide preventative health screenings to their congregations and local communities. If your church does not have a health ministry, suggest creating one. Where there is already such a significant ministry in place, mental health needs to be included.

3. **Preaching and Teaching.** I recall so vividly the first time that I heard a pastor preach on depression and continued what was a monthly teaching series on it. His authenticity and nonjudgmental approach caused at least a hundred members and visitors to respond to his altar call, including me. If more pastors would advocate for mental health from their pulpits, it will help eradicate stigmas and open the door for those hurting within their congregations to reach out for help.

Moving From Victim to Victor

There should be no shame in acknowledging that one is a victim of a traumatic event. There should be no shame in admitting that one is affected by a mental illness either as a side effect from a trauma or because it is the main diagnosis. Victims can become survivors. You can survive a gunshot wound and still be a victim of a drive by shooting. But if you are still mentally held hostage by the incident, you can not live a victorious life. There is a difference in surviving versus overcoming. Survivors become victorious by becoming over comers.

I do not think any healthy person deliberately seeks

to become a victim of anything. Therefore, I believe that all victims desire to become victors. Sometimes there are extenuating external and internal circumstances that enables victims from moving through the appropriate stages. There is a stage that is necessary for one to have a victim's mentality. This concept can be applied to sexual assault or mental illness. When a person initially learns of a diagnosis or have been recently attacked, it is important for them to know that they did not cause their physical, mental or sexual attack. It is also imperative that their victor mentality is mobilized.

When a patient is given crutches due to a bodily injury it is meant to be used as a temporary support mechanism. To ensure that the patient does not become permanently reliant on the crutches, he or she is instructed to participate in some form of physical therapy to assist in gradually weaning them off. Like so, victims have to take the necessary steps in order to be weaned from a victim's mentality. A few disabling tools are anger, bitterness, fear and rejection. A victorious mindset is enabled by hope, faith, positive thinking and positive declarations.

The fifth chapter of Galatians outlines for us the

fruit of the Spirit, as well as, the fruit of the flesh. It is the latter that is least preached about and that hinders the process from moving from a victim's mentality. When fleshly desires take root in our spirit, we give them permission to override what the Spirit desires. I know this to be true. I have had to deal with the war of my fleshly desires and emotions in order to overcome major and even minor trials.

Overcoming to me meant having to overcome myself. It meant dealing with feelings towards others; those I blamed for my circumstances or who I considered to have contributed to them. It meant having the heart to forgive those who did directly contribute to my life's journey even in a negative way. It meant letting go of toxic things even those that had become normal to hold on to. It meant accepting people for who they are while generating healthy boundaries for me. It meant accepting wholeheartedly who I am while believing God's truth.

Have I won the battle of my mind? My answer is yes. As I boldly had to declare in a preaching message during my first engagement after experiencing the episode I described in the *Leading While Bleeding* chapter, "All I Know is What He Said" and the He is referencing God.

Will I have more episodes? Probably. I definitely had many 'come to Jesus' moments while writing this book due to having flashbacks of the incidents described in these memoirs. Does this mean that I am not victorious in my mind or faith? I can firmly state it does not. Victory is my end result that is produced by a daily process. One does not have to walk in fear of what might happen because the Bible unmistakably declares that "For God hath not given us a spirit of fear; but of power, and of love, and of a sound mind" (2 Timothy 1:7, KJV).

As I endeavor to bring a period to this chapter, as well as, this portion of my life's story, I want to briefly share a mental annotation of mine from a renowned film. In the movie, It's a Wonderful Life, the character of George Bailey contemplates suicide when he thinks he has no other options in life to solve his problems. He was able to save himself when he momentarily forgot about his problems in order to help save someone else. When he grasps what the alternative would be if he wasn't alive or never existed; how many people actually cared about him, he realizes that it is indeed a wonderful life!

I have ceased asking God why I had to be one of the ones to bare the thorn of a mental disorder. Bibliology will reveal forerunners of faith that also dealt with this same thorn. In spite of, I could think of so many ways how my life would be less messy. But I thank God for using my mess and making it a message; therefore, using my weaknesses to give strength and encouragement to someone else. The process of keeping my faith while saving my mind means being an advocate and being an ambassador for Christ in order to bridge the gap between faith and mental health. This is my ministry. This is my purpose. This is the journey of my life that I will freely continue to travel with the LORD as my compass.

PRAYER: *Father God, I thank You for the life of the person reading this book and the lives they will touch. LORD, I ask that you will enable their Holy Ghost power so that they might have the strength to overcome and help others become overcomers. Place your Super on their natural so that they might stand against the enemy and break every barrier that hinders healing and deliverance. I decree and declare that stigmas shall be removed, shame shall be exterminated and silence shall be broken. God release your ministry of helps and reconciliation. Regulate minds. Eradicate fears. Mend hearts. Restore relationships. Save the unsaved. Revive the saved. To those that feel as though all hope is gone, remind them of your Word, that mandates they shall not die, but live and declare the works of the Lord.*
In JESUS Name,
Amen.

ABOUT THE AUTHOR

Shulanda J. Hastings, is an evangelist, inspirational writer, novelist and Christian counselor who serves as an Ambassador to the faith-based community; helping to break barriers to healthy relationships and a healthy mind. She is the author of the Beauty of My Thorns novel series, co-author of Letters to America and has authored several devotional books. She is the founder and senior ministry leader of Spirit Realm Divine Manifestation ministries. Shulanda is a native of Clarksdale, Mississippi and currently resides in Memphis, Tennessee.

To connect with author:

Write:
Shulanda J. Hastings
P.O. Box 750041
Memphis, TN 38175
901.606.7792

Email:
Shulanda@sjhastings.com

For blog, books and bookings;
www.ShulandaJHastings.com

Social Media
Facebook: Ambassador Shulanda
Twitter: AmbassadorSJH
Pinterest: Shulandajh
Google+: ShulandaHastingsj7

Endnotes

[i] Clinton, Tim, & Hawkins, Ron. (2009). *The Quick Reference Guide to Biblical Counseling.* Grands Rapid, Michigan. Baker Books.

[ii] Diane Langberg, Ph.D.

[iii] Webster's New World Dictionary. (1996).

[iv] Kubler-Ross, Elisabeth. *On Death and Dying.* (1969)

[v] Mayo Clinic. www.mayoclinic.org (2014).

[vi] National Institute of Mental Health. www.nimh.nih.gov

[vii] Meyer, Joyce. (2011). *Battlefield of the Mind.*

[viii] Merriam-Webster. www.merriam-webster.com

[ix] Corrigan, Patrick W. and Rao, Deepa. (2012). *On the Self-Stigma of Mental Illness: Stages, Disclosure and Strategies for Change.*

[x] National Alliance on Mental Illness (NAMI). www.nami.org

[xi] American Foundation for Suicide Prevention (AFSP). www.afsp.org

[xii] World Health Organization. www.who.in

[xiii] Ibid.

[xiv] Johnson, Brad & Johnson, William. (2014). *The Minister's Guide to Psychological Disorders and Treatments.* 2nd Edition.